Cupping 1

By: Erik Smith

Table Of Contents

Free Stuff

Do you want to get notified when I have free books? Then sign up for my newsletter. I will never spam you. I will only send you valuable stuff that you can use to help you improve your life.

Sign up here - http://forms.aweber.com/form/26/1968511626.htm

Disclaimer

This document is geared towards providing exact and reliable information in regards to the topic and issue covered. The publication is sold with the idea that the publisher is not required to render accounting, officially permitted, or otherwise, qualified services. If advice is necessary, legal or professional, a practiced individual in the profession should be ordered.

- From a Declaration of Principles which was accepted and approved equally by a Committee of the American Bar Association and a Committee of Publishers and Associations.

In no way is it legal to reproduce, duplicate, or transmit any part of this document in either electronic means or in printed format. Recording of this publication is strictly prohibited and any storage of this document is not allowed unless with written permission from the publisher. All rights reserved.

The information provided herein is stated to be truthful and consistent, in that any liability, in terms of inattention or otherwise, by any usage or abuse of any policies, processes, or directions contained within is the solitary and utter responsibility of the recipient reader. Under no circumstances will any legal responsibility or blame be held against the publisher for any reparation, damages, or monetary loss due to the information herein, either directly or indirectly.

Respective authors own all copyrights not held by the publisher.

The information herein is offered for informational purposes solely, and is universal as so. The presentation of the information is without contract or any type of guarantee assurance.

The trademarks that are used are without any consent, and the publication of the trademark is without permission or backing by the trademark owner. All trademarks and brands within this book are for clarifying purposes only and are the owned by the owners themselves, not affiliated with this document.

Introduction

Maybe you've been wondering what those red circles on Michael Phelps' and Jennifer Aniston's backs are. Lately, the spotlight has been shining on this alternative healing method called Cupping Therapy.

What you may not know is that this therapeutic technique was performed by ancient cultures long before Olympic athletes and Hollywood celebrities introduced it to the limelight. Cupping, which is otherwise known as myofascial decompression, is an age-old massage therapy method performed by placing a suction cup-like apparatus on the affected area of a person's body. This is done to create negative pressure to achieve the desired result.

Such results range from providing relief to sore muscles to breaking up post-operative scar tissue. In this book, you will read about the rich history of cupping therapy and follow its journey from the imperial courts of ancient China to the red carpet.

Whether you're a gymnast or a desk worker, there are so many ways in which cupping therapy can benefit you. Find out more about how cupping therapy works and the numerous health benefits that it offers.

Speculations have been raised regarding the safety and effectiveness of cupping therapy. The red bruises alone are enough to make anyone hesitate about engaging in this healing technique. This book's aim is to serve as your complete beginner's guide to cupping therapy and to provide factual, unbiased answers to the frequently asked questions about cupping. Through these pages, you will also become familiarized with the various methods of cupping, the different types of tools used, and other necessary knowledge to maximize the effectiveness and safety of the therapy.

What it is and How it Works

What is Cupping Therapy?

Cupping therapy is a kind of alternative medicine backed by historical reports that can be traced back to 5,000 years in the past. In ancient Chinese medicine, cupping was frequently performed in conjunction with other more well-known alternative healing methods like acupressure and acupuncture.

Basically, cupping therapy is done by arranging cups on the person's skin, directly on top of the body parts that need to be healed. These cups will serve to form a vacuum, which ends up drawing blood to the skin's
surface and to the specific body area that requires healing.

According to ancient belief, all matter is comprised of energy, even your body. A person's state of health depends on the equilibrium of the energies within his body. In order for that balance to be achieved, the energies must be allowed to flow freely within the body and without. This means there must be a free exchange of energies between your body and the environment. This way, you can let go of all the negative energies that you harbor while absorbing the free-floating positive energy around you. In Chinese traditional medicine, there are meridian lines believed to be situated across our bodies. These lines are the pathways though which chi (life energy) travels throughout the body. Chi flows through your blood vessels, your tissues, and your vital organs. When the natural energy pathways in your body are clogged up, this is manifested through physical and mental illnesses.

Think of the meridians as intersections where various roads within the body meet. They connect every organ, every muscle, every cell, and every atom within the body to each other, allowing them to function as one unit.

They link the upper part of your body with the lower part of your body. They connect the internal parts of your body with the external parts of your body. They also serve as the channels through which your feelings and your thoughts, both conscious and subconscious, are communicated throughout the rest of your body. For instance, when your body's temperature is too high, a message is sent to other parts of your body to increase sweat production to help release the heat and thus, cool the body. Likewise, when you perceive a threat, a message is passed throughout the body for the muscles to tense up so you are ready to spring into action.

When something hampers this delicate communication structure, the systems within your body lose their connection with each other and thus become out of sync. As a result, some systems overcompensate while others tend to undercompensate. The organs malfunction and you get sick.

Cupping therapy is based on the theory that when suction is created on specific points of your body, it will assist in drawing out the obstructions. Consequently, it will allow free energy flow through your body systems as well as free energy exchange between your body and the environment. In other words, cupping therapy works by restoring the harmony within your body so it will be in the optimum state to heal itself.

Back in the ancient days, the healers made use of a broad variety of materials for cupping, ranging from the horns and skeletons of animals to bamboo and seashells. These days, cupping therapy is performed with the use of medical standard cups made from materials such as glass, rubber, or silicone. Mechanical pumps are also more popularly used. These cups will be applied on top of the skin right over the painful, diseased, or injured body part. In the most basic method (dry method), a vacuum will be created through heating, followed by immediate cooling of the air within the cups. These cups are left in place for a minimum of five minutes to a maximum of fifteen minutes.

How does cupping therapy work?

Like massage, cupping is a form of deep tissue therapy. One of the biggest differences though is that cupping treatment reaches deeper into the tissues by four inches from the skin's surface. In the dry cupping technique, the bottom part of the cups are rubbed with alcohol. Alternatively, herbs, paper, or a cotton swab saturated with alcohol may be placed inside the cups. Immediately prior to the therapy, these objects are ignited. Just as the flame in the cup dwindles, the practitioner places the cup upside down on the patient's body. As the air cools within the cup, a vacuum is created. This negative pressure dilates the blood vessels situated beneath the skin. As a result, blood flow towards the area is stimulated.

As we get older, the body inevitably breaks down. There is less adhesion in the fascia. You'll notice wrinkles appearing here and there. Muscle loss occurs. There is a noticeable decrease in muscle tone. Blood flow decreases. And with decreased physical activity due to aching joints and fatigue, there is a subsequent decrease in blood supply to the tissues. The tissues covering our muscles and our organs become knotted and misshapen which consequently limits our range of motion even more. It's an ugly cycle that is very real and yet very few people know about it. Thankfully, the reverse pressure created by cupping counteracts this effect.

The suction created in cupping works by directing oxygenated blood towards body areas that need it the most. The tissues become replenished with fresh blood. At the same time, the vacuum works by mobilizing the blood, which has stagnated in that region. As new blood is delivered towards the tissues, a process referred to as neovascularization occurs. In this process, new blood vessels form on their own. These blood vessels will serve to continuously replenish the tissues in that area with oxygen and other vital nutrients. It is for this reason why compared to other forms of deep tissue therapy, the effects of cupping therapy tend to be more long-lasting. Massage triggers blood flow to the area during the treatment but cupping therapy guarantees a steady supply of blood long after the session.

While neovascularization may not occur after several sessions, first-timers can already benefit from another effect of cupping which is called sterile inflammation. We have been programmed by modern medicine to view inflammation in a negative light. However, inflammation is actually a natural process, which is the body's first step towards healing. Inflammation occurs when your body sends out platelets, WBC, and other substances to the injured area to encourage healing. The vacuum created in cupping therapy causes the different tissue layers to separate. As a result, micro tearing takes place. This is no different from the micro traumas that are created when bodybuilders work out. They purposely "injure" the body to trigger regeneration and muscle growth. In cupping, the patient is able to take advantage of the natural healing chemicals that are released towards the site.

After cupping, the patient's muscles are loosened and muscular stiffness is relieved. That's because the fascia are constantly stretched and thus, they are able to regain and retain their flexibility. Cupping therapy is relaxing, both physically and psychologically. It is a great stress-reliever. More than that, it has proven to be helpful in aiding in the treatment of psychological illnesses.

Is cupping safe? What can you expect from cupping therapy?

Cupping therapy was designed to be a non-invasive to a minimally invasive procedure. The practitioner may apply a number of cups on various points all at the same time. Though heat is an essential part of the traditional style of cupping therapy, burning very rarely occurs when cupping is performed by an experienced practitioner. The practitioner may also place an insulation pad on the patient's skin to make burning accidents less likely.

Moreover, you may opt to use silicon suction apparatus if you do not wish to involve flame in the therapy.

In a way, the mechanism involved in cupping therapy is opposite to that of massage therapy. Whereas the latter involves applying pressure against the skin, the former utilizes the vacuum pressure to pull the skin upwards. That said, the therapist may also mobilize the cups across the flesh in a technique not dissimilar to massage. This is known as sliding cupping. In this type of cupping method, the practitioner must avoid passing the cups across bony prominences to prevent injury.

The cupping technique may differ depending on the therapeutic result that needs to be achieved. For instance, wet cupping which involves pricking the skin with needles or making very small cuts with a scalpel, may be performed to rid a patient of tiny amounts of toxins in the blood. When cupping is done in conjunction with acupuncture, needles will be inserted in the individual's skin prior to applying the cups. One possible side effect of these methods of cupping is skin infections due to poorly sanitized tools. It is for this reason why you should get your cupping treatment done by a specialist instead of receiving them in pop-up booths along the road.

Today, cupping therapy is done with strict adherence to the sterile method. This increases the level of safety. Moreover, prior to performing cupping therapy, the equipment are sterilized using heat and high pressure. The cupping site is also prepped for the therapy through massage. For increased comfort, herbal creams and oils may be used. Massage and hydrotherapy are also part of the post-treatment for the dry form of cupping. The reason for this is to minimize the effects of bruising. The telltale red circles acquired after a cupping session is the result of the blood rising up to the surface of the skin. After receiving therapy, you may be sporting these crimson dots for a whole week to ten days. These are normal and are evidence of the expansion of the capillaries beneath the surface of your skin. Note that these red spots are not meant to be painful.

It is common to experience some discomfort in the initial phase of the therapy but the procedure itself should not be painful. If experienced at all, the pain must only temporary and followed by immediate relief. That said, local anesthetics are now being offered by practitioners per patient's request. Swelling is also common as a result of fluids accumulating beneath the skin. You may notice some blisters forming and the healer will explain that this is an indicator of the effectiveness of the treatment in singling out the ailing body part.

As mentioned previously, wet cupping involves pricking. Prior to piercing, the therapist is expected to apply antiseptic on the skin's surface. Because the skin is cut, a bit of pain is expected. Even so, these cuts are meant to be only superficial and are expected to heal within a brief period without causing any scars. In such cases, the practitioner applies antiseptic on the area afterwards and then covers it with a sterile dressing to prevent infection and to speed up the healing process.

People who have experienced receiving cupping therapy report a noticeable increase in the range of motion of the muscles. This is why cupping is extremely popular among athletes. When used as a form of massage, it can be performed to warm up the muscles before a game or to help reduce muscular tension after an event.

Who is eligible for receiving cupping therapy?

Almost anyone can enjoy the benefits of cupping therapy. That said, it is not recommended for women who are pregnant and ladies who are on their period. Refrain from obtaining this treatment if you have skeletal fractures or if you're suffering from muscular spasms. Do not attempt to have this treatment done if you have high fever accompanied by convulsions.

Cupping therapy is not endorsed to cancer patients due to the risk of spreading the cancer to other areas of the body. If you are taking blood-thinning drugs or supplements or if you're suffering from any medical condition which causes you to bleed easily, cupping therapy may not be for you.

During the session, make sure to tell your therapist to avoid areas of the body, which show signs of deep vein thrombosis. This includes pain and swelling in the calves, a red patch situated at the back of the legs just below the knees, or a clot beneath the skin that's warm to touch. The cups must not be applied on pulse points. They should never be placed directly on top of ulcers.

Individuals who are very skinny are not good candidates for this treatment. As mentioned, the effects of cupping can penetrate the body up to four inches from the skin's surface. Thus, to perform this treatment on thin clients would mean risking injury to the bones or burning of the tissue. Cupping therapy is also not a practical treatment for obese individuals though it can assist in weight loss.

Where it All Begun

Apart from the fact that the practice is thousands of years old, another amazing thing about cupping therapy is its universality. Historical records reveal that this ancient healing technique has been used for treating illnesses and for promoting wellness by various cultures from the Far East to the Western world. Each culture has its own unique name, style, and tools used for cupping. Even so, the process is generally the same. For instance, what was known to the ancient Japanese as Kyukaku was known to the Arabs as Hijama. Several centuries after, we came to know cupping in health spas as the Ventosa. Other names for cupping therapy are as follows:

· Bentousa
· Catacion
· Kuppareita
· Ventuze
· Sang Pori
· Singhi
· Vacuum Therapy
· Kuppaus
· Jiaofa (Horn Technique)
· Txhuav
· Seljale

Cupping in China

Cupping therapy has always been a vital part of Traditional Chinese Medicine. In fact, the most complete accounts of cupping therapy came from ancient China where it was believed to have been practiced 3,000 years ago. The medicine men of ancient China would place hollowed animal horns on acupuncture points because they believed that it would help mobilize stagnated blood and Chi. This would benefit not just the area directly below the animal horn but also the body organ which is linked to that acupuncture point.

This treatment was often given to high-ranking officials in the Chinese imperial courts as part of their privilege.

A Taoist by the name of Ge Hong is known in the world of Traditional Chinese Medicine for his manuscript, A Handbook of Prescriptions for Emergencies. In the book, he wrote about the use of animal horns fashioned into cups to drain pus out of wounds and to draw off negative energy from a person's meridian points.

Another book authored by Wang Tayr of the Tang Dynasty talked about the use of fire cupping methods to help relieve symptoms of headache and stomach pains. During this era, cupping was used hand in hand with acupuncture and moxibustion (burning of medicinal herb mugwort) to treat serious illnesses such as pulmonary tuberculosis.

In the Qing dynasty, in a book written by Zhao Xuemin, liquid cupping therapy was referred to as Ja Qui. In this method, cups were fashioned out of bamboo or clay. These cups are sterilized through boiling and then soaked in herbal solutions. The healer would pierce the affected area with acupuncture needles and then place the cups on the patient's flesh. The medicine folk in those times utilized Ja Qui to treat a broad range of illnesses from common colds to painful joints.

During the 50's, cupping therapy was rendered in Chinese hospitals as an official form of treatment. Today, cupping is still widely used in China and though glass and plastic cups have taken the place of animal horns and earthenware, the key techniques remain the same. Moreover, the government of China is currently expending resources to further the study of the ancient documents and to fund more research to determine the treatment's efficacy.

From the Egyptians to the Persians

The exact first origins of cupping therapy remains unknown. Nevertheless, the images of cupping apparatus in the Ebers Papyrus, an unearthed manuscript dating back to 1550 BCE, made it clear that the ancient Egyptians were no strangers to this healing technique. In fact, the healers in ancient Egypt used cupping as a remedy for just about every ailment in the human body. Back then, they believed that drawing blood from the body and sucking it out would aid in the removal of unnatural substances that cause disease.

The ancient Greeks inherited this medical knowledge from the ancient Egyptians. Hippocrates promoted the use of cupping therapy to cure sicknesses and to boost wellness. Galen was also a firm advocate of the treatment. And in his writings, Herodotus enumerated the following benefits of Cucurbits (cupping):

- Reduces pain in the head
- Reduces inflammation
- Strengthens the digestive system
- Restores appetite
- Treats dizziness
- Draws toxins to the surface
- Dries excess fluids
- Stops bleeding
- Promotes menstrual flow
- Prevents infection
- Shortens the duration of illness
- Gets rid of excess weight
- Treats muscular rigidity
- Treats depression

This medical knowledge was passed on to the Alexandrians and the Byzantines and then later on, to the Romans. After which, the Muslim Arabs and the Persians got hold of this secret wisdom. The Prophet Mohammad himself approved of this form of treatment. In fact, today, cupping therapy is a vital part of the Persian-Arabic Traditional Medicine known as Unani Medicine.

Cupping All Over the World

Perhaps one of the reasons why the concept of cupping is astonishingly universal is because the idea is so basic that it appeals to every man's common sense, regardless of his geographical location or what era he exists in.

Everyone would agree that if something that's in your body should not be there, then it must be removed. Back in ancient times, people from various parts of Asia from China and Japan to Vietnam and Korea used the horns of native beasts to perform cupping because it was the material that was readily available to them. The same is true of African natives. The Indians in North America made use of buffalo horns. Meanwhile, the natives around the Vancouver Island and along the west coast utilized shells for suction cups because they built dwellings near the sea. The people of ancient Babylon and Assyria used skeleton tubes as suction equipment. In the Mediterranean, a form of cupping massage was done by creating suction directly with the mouth.

Cups made of shells or horns are fashioned by cutting off the point of the shell or the horn. The base of the horn or the shell is placed against the body while the practitioner's lips would be pursed around the hole at the tip.
He or she would suck in to create a vacuum. At the same time, the healer may or may not blow a wad of dried herbs through the hole using his or her tongue. From this, you can tell that one of the requirements of medicine men and women at that time was to have flexible facial muscles and an agile tongue.

The Decline and the Rise of Cupping Therapy

Cupping continued to be a popular form of alternative therapy until modern medicine pushed it further and further into the background.

Throughout the centuries, women have always been valued as healers in various cultures. From Russia and Holland to Turkey and Vietnam, cupping therapy was commonly performed by female healers. Female folk healers would pass down the knowledge of cupping therapy from one generation to another. The decline of cupping therapy began when women were denied the right to higher education and were prohibited from sharing their wisdom with male practitioners. At the dawn of the 13th century, schools which taught medicine as part of their curriculum prohibited womenfolk from attending classes. Inevitably, the number of women who were knowledgeable in traditional treatment dwindled. This carried on

well until the early 1800's. During those times, cupping therapy received so much scrutiny and was shunned by the recently established model of medicine.
One needs to understand that the creators of this model made it their goal to discredit all forms of traditional medicine so as to achieve dominance in the medical field.

In the 1960's-70's, Foucalt redefined modern medicine with his "Clinical Gaze" which suggested dehumanizing the patient by treating his body separately from his identity. Since cupping therapy involves treating the body from the surface, it was not congruent with the popular new archetype. Simply put, the reason why cupping therapy suffered from so much opposition was not because of the lack of evidence of its effectiveness. Rather, it was due to the fact that it does not fit perfectly with the new models that the medical community were promoting. In other words, cupping was not compatible with the financial interests of the big corporations who were running the show.

In the advent of the 20th century, cupping therapy certainly lost its popularity in Anglo-Saxon communities. Nevertheless, a surgeon in the 1800's by the name of Charles Kennedy attested to the effectiveness of cupping therapy. This was evidence that the power of cupping therapy may have been temporarily obscured but not totally forgotten. When the Medical Registration Act of 1858 was established, the public's opinion on traditional forms of medical therapy were severely affected and "unofficial" therapeutic methods such as cupping received so much social stigma.

Even so, in the past 20 years, as the negative side effects of pharmaceuticals become more and more apparent, more and more people began embracing alternative methods of medicine. People are looking for ways to free themselves from the colossal destructive machine that is the pharmaceutical industry, a machine that swallows patients up and then spits them out in far worse conditions than when they came in. The tide has certainly turned. More individuals are doing their research and striving to restore the control of their own health back into their hands. With this enlightenment comes the rediscovery of effective, safe, non-invasive, and cost-effective traditional healing practices like cupping therapy. And with the attention drawn by celebrities such as Gwyneth Paltrow and NFL player DeMarcus Ware, one can tell that cupping therapy has certainly risen from the ashes.

Today, holistic practitioners are offering new variations of this ancient healing practice as they start combining it with modern medical knowledge.

How it Can Help You

So much online buzz was created when Michael Phelps tweeted a photo of himself with suction cups all over his buttocks. Now fans know that cupping therapy is part of the swimmer's secret to success. According to a report from the Journal of Traditional and Complementary Medicine dated 2015, cupping therapy is effective in reversing facial paralysis and in pain management. It is also useful in the management of herpes zoster and cervical spondylitis. Moreover, cupping therapy works as a cure for acne and eczema where some medications have failed.

The British Cupping Society states that cupping therapy is beneficial in the treatment of various illnesses from migraines to bronchitis to sore throat. It has also shown effectiveness in addressing inflammatory conditions such as arthritis. In women, cupping therapy aids in promoting fertility and in curing gynecological diseases. Individuals who receive cupping therapy regularly also report to have lower blood pressure. When done on a regular basis, cupping can aid in the treatment of blood disorders ranging from anemia to hemophilia.

Cupping therapy is an effective and holistic means of prettifying yourself.

This traditional treatment is not just used for curing medical conditions but also as a beauty treatment. One of the reasons why it's such a hit among Hollywood celebs is that it aids in facial rejuvenation and visibly decreases facial lines caused by aging. At the same time, it lessens the appearance of varicose veins. Another desired effect of cupping therapy is weight loss. It is also useful in eliminating cellulites. For this purpose, the practitioner will first apply oil onto the patient's skin and then create suction. After which, the cup will be mobilized across the surrounding areas of the receiver's body. Some people also engage in cupping therapy to get rid of scars.

Cupping therapy detoxifies the body and boosts the immune system.

When done regularly, this therapy can minimize the occurrence of seasonal allergies and the common cold.

Cupping therapy leads to a healthier heart.

The wet cupping method is effective in lowering the levels of LDL especially in males. It is a great preventative measure against atherosclerosis.

Cupping therapy is a safe way to alleviate pain.

Unlike pain relievers, cupping does not encourage dependency. It has proven to be effective in eliminating pain from various parts of the body from the head, down to the back, and all the way to the lower extremities. Wet cupping is recommended for individuals suffering from persistent low back pain and carpal tunnel syndrome.

When done in conjunction with acupuncture, cupping therapy can be used to get rid of toothaches. Meanwhile, massage cupping is effective against muscular stiffness. For soft tissue injuries, cupping therapy is implemented in conjunction with plum blossom acupuncture to help manage pain.

Cupping therapy aids in digestive health.
It is believed to be effective in treating a variety of gastrointestinal disorders from diarrhea to gastritis. Kids suffering from mild cases of indigestion may also benefit from cupping therapy.

Cupping therapy promotes mental wellness.
Individuals who receive cupping therapy are less prone to suffering from depression and anxiety. People who seek this traditional therapy often do so for the purpose of relieving stress. Moreover, if you're having trouble with sleeping, this ancient form of therapy just might work for you.

Other health issues resolved by regular wet cupping include genital ulcers and acute conjunctivitis. Meanwhile, the dry cupping technique is known to be more efficient in treating asthma. The next chapter will provide you with a more detailed discussion of the various cupping methods and their indications.

More Stuff You Need to Know Before Receiving Cupping Therapy

Before looking for a practitioner, it is important that you learn more about the different cupping methods, how they are done, and which health problems they are indicated for. This way, you'll have an idea as to which method will work best for you and which technique you'll be most comfortable with.

Dry Cupping

This is the most basic of all cupping techniques. Aside from the method described in the first chapter, the practitioner may simply hold the cups over a small flame so that the air inside them are heated. Afterwards, he/she will place the inverted cups on your skin. Glass cups are usually preferred for this method because this allows the therapist to watch the effect on your skin and thus, burning will easily be prevented. Glass cups also provide the best seal and suction and are more durable than most pressure equipment. At the same time, they are easier to sterilize.

Dry cupping therapy is indicated for the treatment of respiratory conditions. A series of five therapies are usually done to address neck pain. When used to treat knee osteoarthritis, a pulsatile cupping device is used to carry out this method. Dry cupping therapy is also the method of choice for relieving chest pains. Furthermore, it is recommended in combating lethargy in patents who have suffered from cerebrovascular accident.

Massage Cupping

Massage cupping is a subcategory that falls under dry cupping. Another name for it is gliding cupping. In this method, oils are first applied onto the skin and then the heated cups are glided across the patient's body in a sort of reverse massage therapy. This is the method of choice for clients who want to lose weight. It is also effective in getting rid of cellulites. The best type of cupping equipment for this process are medical standard silicone cups or rubber cups. This is because if suction cups are to be moved easily to and fro, they'll need to be softer and more flexible than glass.

Wet Cupping

In this method, the practitioner initially performs dry cupping for about three minutes. Then, he/she makes use of a sterilized blade to create minute cuts on the patient's skin. Another clean cup is placed on the area to siphon the drops of blood. This is the technique used when a patient wants to get rid of drugs, venom, and other foreign substances from the body. Afterwards, an antibiotic ointment is applied and the site is wrapped in sterile bandages. In the traditional Chinese technique, thick gauge needles with three edges are used for creating the punctures. This method is indicted for treating facial paralysis, dermatitis, and periauricular pain.

In Al Hijama, a detoxifying cupping method performed in Islamic cultures, the incisions are created on a spot on the patient's back, situated between the shoulder blades and the neck. This is usually done around the 17th, the 19th, and the 21st days of the Muslim lunar calendar.

BLC

Sometimes, wet cupping is referred to as BLC (bloodletting cupping). There are many variations of BLC. When used in the treatment of gouty arthritis and rheumatoid arthritis, it is performed in combination with herbal drugs. For treating soft tissue injuries, Chinese plum blossom needles are preferred. Meanwhile, when used for the treatment of acne, the piercing is done first and then a facial mask is applied. For cases of neurodermatitis, red hot needles are used.

Air Cupping

This method is also popularly known as vacuum cupping. In this method, heat and fire are not necessary so it's ideal for beginners. In this technique, a pump is affixed to the upper part of the cup and the practitioner manually pumps air out in order to form a vacuum. After the desired amount of suction has been reached, the therapist seals the valve located on top of the cup and then disconnects the pumping apparatus. As you can see, one of the benefits of this method is that the specialist has more control over the amount of suction that is delivered, thus lessening the risk of discomfort and injury.

Prior to the session, the therapist cleanses the site and massages the patient's skin with a lubricant such as an herbal oil. The suction tools and cups are usually cleansed in warm saline solution.
After five to fifteen minutes, the therapist then opens the valve to remove the vacuum and then he/she detaches the cups gently from the skin. Sometimes, blisters may appear after the therapy. These contain accumulated toxic fluids. With the consent of the patient, the practitioner will prick these blisters so that the contaminated blood will be eliminated. In this case, air cupping becomes a form of wet cupping.

Face Cupping

As you may have probably guessed, facial cupping is performed to aid in improving the facial skin. It is done to get rid of wrinkles, dark circles around the eyes, acne scars, and even sagging flesh and double chins. More than that, face cupping has proven to be effective in treating migraines, sinusitis, stiff mandibles, and earaches. In individuals with Parkinson's disease, face cupping helps in reducing the impact of facial paralysis. Some patients receive face cupping therapy to get rid of facial tics as well as undesirable and uncontrollable facial mannerisms.

Before the procedure, the therapist applies herbal creams or oils all over the patient's face and neck area. The special glass cups used in face cupping are affixed to rubber bulbs which serve as manual pumps for generating mild suction. The practitioner then glides the cups along the facial skin, the neck, and even the chest. The purpose of this is to trigger the rush of oxygenated blood and nutrients into the facial area. This activates the formation of collagen. The result? Noticeably supple facial skin with a healthy glow. The advantage of face cupping technique over other forms of cupping is that it does not leave red marks on the face.

Acupuncture Cupping

In this method, wet cupping is performed along with acupuncture. After injecting needles into pressure points, the heated cups are lain on top of the selected sites. This is the method of choice for ankylosing spondylitis and fibromyalgia. Meanwhile, mild pressure cupping combined with laser acupuncture are best for treating pain in the lower back. When combined with BLC and gliding cupping, acupuncture cupping can be used to treat chloasma.

Water Cupping

This Islamic technique of cupping is probably the most dangerous of all the methods. Therefore, it should only be done by licensed practitioners. It is performed by adding warm water into the cups. A ball of flaming cotton ball is thrown into the cups and then each cup is arranged inversely on the patient's skin. Experienced water cupping therapists are able to do this without spilling even a drop of water. This is the method of choice for treating high fever related to infections of the respiratory tract.

Whichever cupping method you choose, it is necessary that you seek a trained cupping therapist. Such therapists carry licenses to perform cupping. A certified practitioner will screen patients thoroughly prior to performing therapy. He or she will gather your baseline data and your medical history and will assess if cupping is safe for you. Moreover, the professional cupping therapist will perform the treatment in a secure and sterile environment using medically approved and disinfected instruments. This is crucial especially if wet cupping or BLC are to be administered. Remember that reusing needles and scalpels can place you at risk for acquiring blood-borne diseases like AIDS. A licensed practitioner of wet cupping or BLC also has knowledge on how to dress wounds and will provide you with appropriate post-care instructions. Furthermore, note that only qualified therapists are authorized to administer anesthetics. Individual cupping therapy sessions cost somewhere from $30 to $80, depending on the kind of method used.

Conclusion

Thank you again for downloading this book!

I hope this book was able to help you understand the concept of cupping therapy and how it can aid in improving your overall physical and mental health.
Regain control over your health and wellbeing. Take your freedom back from money-making pharmaceutical companies and the modern medical industry.

The next step is to decide for yourself whether cupping therapy is the right treatment for you. This book has provided you with all the facts and now it's up to you to decide which approach to take concerning your health and your life.

Finally, if you enjoyed this book, then I'd like to ask you for a favor, would you be kind enough to leave a review for this book on Amazon? It'd be greatly appreciated!

Thank you and good luck!

Free Stuff

Do you want to get notified when I have free books? Then sign up for my newsletter. I will never spam you. I will only send you valuable stuff that you can use to help you improve your life.

Sign up here - http://forms.aweber.com/form/26/1968511626.htm

Made in the USA
Middletown, DE
14 July 2017